DOG TRAINING

A Step-by-step Guide to Teach Your Dog

(A Beginner's Guide to Dog Training for all breeds)

Vernon Moore

Published by Harry Barnes

Vernon Moore

All Rights Reserved

Dog Training: A Step-by-step Guide to Teach Your Dog (A Beginner's Guide to Dog Training for all breeds)

ISBN 978-1-77485-161-6

All rights reserved. No part of this guide may be reproduced in any form without permission in writing from the publisher except in the case of brief quotations embodied in critical articles or reviews.
Legal & Disclaimer

The information contained in this book is not designed to replace or take the place of any form of medicine or professional medical advice. The information in this book has been provided for educational and entertainment purposes only.

The information contained in this book has been compiled from sources deemed reliable, and it is accurate to the best of the Author's knowledge; however, the Author cannot guarantee its accuracy and validity and cannot be held liable for any errors or omissions. Changes are periodically made to this book. You must consult your doctor or get professional medical advice before using any of the suggested remedies, techniques, or information in this book.

Upon using the information contained in this book, you agree to hold harmless the Author from and against any damages, costs, and expenses, including any legal fees potentially resulting from the application of any of the information provided by this guide. This disclaimer applies to any damages or injury caused by the use and application, whether directly or indirectly, of any advice or information presented, whether for breach of contract, tort, negligence, personal injury, criminal intent, or under any other cause of action.

You agree to accept all risks of using the information presented inside this book. You need to consult a professional medical practitioner in order to ensure you are both able and healthy enough to participate in this program.

Table of Contents

INTRODUCTION 1

CHAPTER 1: BUILDING A RELATIONSHIP WITH AN OBEDIENT PUPPY 4

CHAPTER 2: HOW TO TRAIN YOUR DOG TO BE A GUARD DOG 10

CHAPTER 3: THE ESSENTIAL THINGS TO CONSIDER BEFORE YOU START PUPPY TRAINING 17

CHAPTER 4: TRAINING TO THE NICKNAME 24

CHAPTER 5: BRINGING YOUR PUPPY HOME FOR THE FIRST TIME 38

CHAPTER 6: WHY IS DOG TRAINING IMPORTANT? 52

CHAPTER 7: GET TO KNOW YOUR DOG 57

CHAPTER 8: BASICS OF DOG TRAINING 72

CHAPTER 9: UNDERSTANDING YOUR DOG'S NEEDS IS KEY 77

CHAPTER 10: HOW DO YOU TRAIN YOUR DOG? 83

CHAPTER 11: THE BASIC COMMANDS 89

CHAPTER 12: STARTING YOUR PUPPY OFF ON THE RIGHT PAW 96

CHAPTER 13: PUPPY TRAINING FOR NEW DOG OWNERS 99

CHAPTER 14: HAVANEDZE TRAINING WHAT TO DO IF YOUR DOG HAS SEVERE ANXIETY 111

CHAPTER 15: HOUSEBREAKING YOUR PUPPY IN 4 EASY STEPS 122

CHAPTER 16: PUPPY PROOFING YOUR HOUSE 127

CHAPTER 17: HOW TO TEACH YOUR DOG ADVANCED SKILLS 132

CONCLUSION 143

Introduction

Dog owners have been training their dogs for as long as they can remember. There are many benefits to training your dog. Caesar Millan, a canine behavior expert, says that training your dog will benefit both you and your dog. It will allow your dog to discover their natural talents and skills. This will also help you to bond with your dog through the sharing of new tricks. Teaching a dog tricks can have many benefits, not only for your mental health but also for your pet's physical well-being.
Engaging your dog in agility or fetch training will allow them to live a more active, free lifestyle. This is more like how they would act in the wild. According to the American Kennel Club, dogs that are engaged in physical activity can help prevent many diseases.

This book will teach you twenty-five tricks that even someone with no training experience can learn. You can learn to call your dog to come, sit or stay on command. Or you can do something more fun like a barking command or army crawl.

Before you start training your dog, I suggest you buy treats and a clicker for your dog. Even an old dog can learn new tricks. I hope you and your dog will strengthen your already strong relationship by learning the tricks in this book. Remember that these techniques are not for dogs. You must also be patient.

You teach your dog that consistency and repetition are important. For a command to be effective, you must repeat the same word every time (e.g. You must use the same word for each command (e.g., "sit" or "stay")

For each command you must use the exact same hand motion (e.g. For "stay", raise your palm and point two fingers to the ground with your fingers.

You must practice every day with your dog the trick or tricks that you have taught him the previous day. Start with a simple trick like "sit", and once he's performing the task correctly, you can go back to that command for your next practice session. This will ensure that he is competent and that he knows how to do it. You should praise your dog for every successful trick. You can reward your dog with a treat, such as a green bean, raw baby carrot or dog cookie.

You and your dog can work together if you are consistent and adhere to these rules. Your dog will be happy and well-behaved if you're consistent.

Chapter 1: Building a relationship with an Obedient Puppy

You've made the decision to add a puppy into your family. This is one of your best decisions. A dog can help reduce stress in the family, and it will teach your children how to be more responsible.

A dog can be a family member, and it will also provide a companion that can perform certain tasks, entertain you, and protect you against any outsiders.

This puppy is still small, but it will grow into a fully grown dog in just a few months. It is impossible to predict what you will get from each puppy or dog that you adopt. You could get a dominant alpha or beta type dog. If you are lucky, tey might even become an omega. It is in your best interests to be able control your dog at all time and expect obedience.

These are the reasons why so many dog training schools make huge profits today.

Did you know you can train your dog efficiently by using a few tips also shared by experts? It is impossible to expect a dog with a military-grade obedience level. You can ensure your dog knows what to do when you call. This will take patience and time, but you will be grateful and have a long, enjoyable relationship with your dog. Before we get started, there are some things to keep in mind when you're considering getting a dog or puppy.

Breed

There are many breeds of dog, each with its own personality and temperament. People often buy a dog just because they like its appearance, without considering whether it will suit their personalities. If you have a busy family and can't devote enough time to caring for a dog like a Siberian Husky or German Shepherd, then you will end up with a dog who is bored and has a lot of energy. If you are a fitness buff and enjoy running, you shouldn't expect your Maltese to keep up with you as you run long distances.

Before you buy a dog, do your research to ensure that you're a good match. Although you may not find the ideal dog, you will have a stronger relationship with your pet over time.

Energy level

This is also an important consideration for breeds. Different breeds of dog have different energy levels. It is important to choose a dog with the same energy level that you do. You could also find one you can exercise with enough to burn off the excess energy.

High-energy dogs work best for athletes and people who are physically active. These dogs are great for work and have an inexhaustible supply of energy. These dogs can run for up to an hour, so they'll have fun outside.

A mild-mannered, low-energy dog is a great match for families with children and elderly people. They are gentle and easy to train and will not harm anyone. Although they still require some exercise, this will not be as much as working dogs. They will be content to lay down at the feet of their masters after a quick 15-minute stroll around the block.

There are also dogs who can be relegated to being couch potatoes, which are great for people who are too busy or absent for long periods of the day, or who are physically or mentally unable or too tired to walk their dog.

It is important to find a dog who matches your energy level.

Family Dynamics

When choosing a dog, it is important to consider your family dynamics. There are many kinds of families today. There is usually one dominant member of a family that is more dominant than all others. Your family will be your dog's pack. Find out who this is. Before you bring your dog in as the Omega, make sure to determine who will be the Alpha and Beta of the pack. Your dog should not be acting as the Alpha, with you and your family being relegated into Beta or Omega.

Chapter 2: How to train your dog to be a guard dog

Dog owners are keen to train their dogs. The majority can teach their dogs basic tricks such as sitting and playing dead. Some dog owners want their dogs to be friends with everyone, especially their immediate family. Dog owners would like their dogs to be trained for protection. This is why many people get a dog as a pet.

They would be kept safe in their home, or they could bark if there is a danger.

Dog owners who lack the time or difficulty to train their dogs can have problems with personal security. It's not easy to get your dog to sit or fetch, so imagine how difficult it will be to train your dog for security. Are you ever wishing you could teach your dog to be alert and defend you when you are in need? This is what you can do.

Dog owners often settle for basic training because it is easier to do.

Some dogs are easier to train than others. Others have the natural ability and skill to understand their owners and comply with them. Proper dog training is the best way to make sure that your dog is well-trained and safe.

You can train your dog to be a guardian or to protect yourself. However, it's possible to train your dog by hiring a professional trainer.

TECHNIQUES TO TRAIN YOUR DOG IN PERSONAL PROTECTION

Teach your dog obedience.

To train your dog to be obedient, the first step is to teach it how to listen. You must teach your dog to obey basic commands such as sit, stay, stop and bark. One way to determine if your dog is ready to become a guardian dog is to train him or her to obey commands. Use positive feedback to encourage your dog to continue the training.

This will help your dog to be more responsive and willing to learn from you. Because he knows that he will be rewarded for doing the right thing, he will also be more submissive.

LEAVE YOUR DOG TO VISIT THE ENVIRONMENT IN WHICH THEY LIVE.

Allow your dog to have a chance to meet other dogs so that he can learn to judge them. This will help them to distinguish between a dangerous person and a nice one. The dog is able to perceive and respond faster to environmental factors. Your dog can be familiarized with his family members so that he knows who he should guard. Your dog can see you doing your daily activities to help him distinguish it from an unusual event.

TEACH YOUR DOG HOW TO BARK

Your dog should be allowed to bark at strangers. It is best to teach your dog to bark at strangers. If you can get them to stop barking, they should obey your commands. Two common signs that a dog barks at others are: The dog barks when he sees a dog he likes or when he feels threatened. Although barking is a natural behavior for dogs, it's important to be able teach your dog when to stop barking.

Tell your dog to go hide from his friends and family members, then knock on the doors or windows. If your dog makes this unusual sound when barking, it's a sign that he is learning how and when to bark. Your dog shouldn't bark at anyone, not even your family members, unless you ask him to or if there isn't danger. If your dog can't stop barking at you, it might not be a good choice for personal protection.

This article will help you make it easier to communicate with your dog.

TEACH YOUR DOG TO NOT EAT FOOD FROM STRANGERS

This is important as hoodlums will use this strategy to get along with the dog. You can allow them to have free access to your home without being disturbed. Your family members or friends who visit the dog once in a while should not feed it. You can do the feeding or ask someone else to do it. So that your dog is able to trust you with food, it is better to let your entire family access your home. This will help your dog to know who to eat and not.

TEACH YOUR DOG TO DEFEND, AND NOT TO ATTACK

Remember that your goal is to train your dog as a personal protector and not an attack dog. It is very different to teach your dog how to defend you from attacking.

He wouldn't be allowed to bite someone you happen to meet at the recreation center. Dogs that have been trained to attack others are dangerous to keep as pets. Dogs have been known to attack a significant portion of their owners relatives. This is not something you want to have happen to your dog. You should teach your dog to obey you and to attack only when instructed. Personal protection is not possible with dogs that are too forceful or aggressive and who attack people without being instructed.

Chapter 3: The Essential Things to Consider Before You Start Puppy Training

A new puppy was brought home and everyone is happy for him to join the family. The puppy will be captivated by the excitement around him.

He will adapt to his environment as you taught him. To achieve this level of performance, you will need a puppy training method. This technique is available if you wish.

But I will show you the 4 best basic techniques.

Many people are concerned about their dog pooping in their homes. Puppy's don't come with any potty training and will poo wherever they want to. The puppy training method will determine how much you and your family will love the puppy.

This form of discipline is not meant to be used as punishment. Instead, treat the puppy like your child. Your puppy will be more comfortable if you pay attention to them than if they are recognized. They will want to impress you by being praised. This is open to horses and children.

If you let your puppies become dogs, it is impossible to train them. These are the easy strategies that you can use in order to succeed.

Bravo! You need to know when your dog is going to have to go potty. Every puppy knows when it is time to go. These signals are what they need.

This is the foundational preparation. This training involves teaching him how to sit, stand, and kneel. To make him quickly understand, be consistent.

Your family members should participate in the class. You must remind them to use this term to avoid complicating matters. Don't stretch your puppy, let your family know. Loyalty is key here as it is what drives them to learn quickly.

It is important to be able to communicate with your dog when it is time to do his thing. You can take your puppy with you at any time during the day, whenever it is convenient for him. You should clearly indicate where and when you will feed your puppy.

After you have finished feeding your baby, take him to the toilet at least once an hour. This helps them understand their routines and schedule.

Crate teaching - Let him know the value of the crate. You can take the crate with you when you go shopping, or on a vacation.

Humans need to be patient. This quality is often lacking in many people. This is an essential quality for puppy training.

It is because you will need to spend a lot of time before you see results. This can be frustrating. Although it may not seem like a difficult task, puppy training is actually quite hard.

Puppy training is a continuous process. To see the first results, you must practice it consistently. Before the puppy can learn each command, he must first understand what it means.

To train your puppy to be a good dog, you will need patience and a lot of time. Your puppy might not understand all of your instructions the first few days.

You will lose patience if you don't have enough patience. Your puppy will see this and decide you want to play with him. This will frustrate even more. This is a sign that you need to end your training session and start the next one.

You can take steps to avoid getting frustrated. You can think about the fact that learning new things can be frustrating if you are feeling frustrated.

Your puppy is still a puppy. You can train your puppy with a lot of effort and hard work.

Your puppy will not be able to understand you, but he might understand your emotions. Your puppy will sense when you are upset and will play with you or roll over to cheer you up.

This will only make things worse. If you are unable to calm down, it is best to end the day and resume puppy training the next day.

You may consider hiring a professional if you are not patient enough or feel unable to manage puppy training. You will reap the benefits of a trained dog and not have to work for it.

You could also opt to not get a puppy or train an older dog. A puppy may not be the best choice for you if you lack patience. Because a puppy must be trained in patience at least for the first year.

How to tell if your puppy needs formal training

Ownership of a marionette can be a huge responsibility. Therefore, it is important to get marionette training started as soon as possible. This is where the question comes in: How can you tell if your dog can be taught or if he prefers formal training?

Some dogs respond faster to training than others, and some puppies still struggle to master commands even with the best home trainer. These dogs will benefit from intensive obedience training. Your trainer will focus on your puppy's problems and help you solve them.

Some dogs are more responsive to humans than others, even if they have never been raised. You are very fortunate to have a puppy who does this. The majority of animals are not like that. Your puppy is not a wild animal. This is just a sign that your puppy needs to be taught how to perform properly in public.

This formal training will teach your dog basic obedience commands as well as how to react when strangers approach. For any problems you may have with your puppy after you bring him home, we recommend formal training.

You can also determine if your pet requires intensive puppy training by looking at your calendar. You must also consider the cost of lessons, as they can be expensive.

You don't have to prepare if they don't work out. It may take longer but it will be the best for your family. It is not worth spending money on things you don't need.

Puppy school is a good option if you are unable to teach your dog by yourself. Dogs learn the most when they follow a schedule. Your puppy will forget what you did and start over again if you are absent for more than a week.

There are many things to keep in mind when you train your dog. It is important to decide if you want to train your puppy at home or in a class. Also, it is important to follow your plan.

Chapter 4: Training to the Nickname

Nicknames are short, evocative words that do not include the names of people, cities, countries, or nationalities. The conditional reflex to the nickname develops during daily dog-handling, but is more common when a dog is walked or fed.

The trainer (the owner) calls the dog and tells him the nickname. He then gives the dog food or treats. The dog will pay more attention to the nickname as it begins to walk and learn techniques to train. It is not acceptable to use a frightening tone of voice or to incite fear.

Trainer faults and the implications

1. A mispronunciation of nickname, especially when it is sounded menacing.

2. It is not necessary to repeatedly repeat a nickname. This can hinder the formation of conditional reflexes on other commands.

Training for Special Equipment

Training is usually done at an early age for muzzle, collar, and leash dogs. They are taught to be calm around the collar. The trainer will then give the dog a treat and allow them to sniff the collar. After stroking the dog with his hands, the trainer wraps the collar around the neck of the dog and holds the ends in play to distract it. The collar can be removed if the dog is having trouble. The exercise is then repeated. The collar should be left on for longer periods of time. The soft collar can then be replaced with the normal. It is important to make sure that the puppies do not chew each other's collars if there are several of them.

After training the dog to calmly respond to the collar, it is time to train the dog to use a leash. The trainer strokes the dog and then attaches the leash.

It is important to play a game with your dog or to keep it from reacting to the leash. Dog management in areas where there are trees, shrubs, or other obstructions is a delicate task. Short and long leashes are used for dog management.

The size of the dog's head determines the muzzle. The trainer will be watching the dog while he walks it or takes care of him. He will place a piece of treat in the muzzle and issue the command "Muzzle." This allows the dog to get a treat as well as eat, and encourages the dog by stroking. The muzzle should be tucked in and the dog must follow the instructions. The trainer will distract the dog by playing, running, or giving it a treat through its muzzle hole if the dog attempts to remove the muzzle. It's okay to have a muzzle on for 5-10 minutes at first. Then, the muzzle can be worn for a while.

Trainer faults and the implications

1. The wrong equipment can increase the amount of time it takes to train a dog.

2. Prematurely increasing the time the dog is wearing the equipment by using painful stimuli can lead to fear of the trainer.

3. Uncontrollable play with a dog's leash can lead to a habit of biting at the leash.

The Command "Come!"

After being given a command or seeing a gesture, the dog must immediately come to the trainer. This skill teaches the dog to be more attentive to their trainer and discipline them.

The command, "Come!" The command "Come!" and the gesture: lowering your left hand to your thighbone.

Reinforcement – Give the treat, stroke and sometimes tighten your leash.

It is started from the day the dog starts walking. Dog training begins with food.

Training is conducted in an area that has the fewest distractions. The dog should be hungry, or half-starved, and be able to walk well. This is how the exercise is done. The trainer calls the dog's name, draws attention to the meat in his left hand, and then commands him to "Come!" The thumb keeps the treat in the hand. The hand should move freely at first. Next, raise the left hand and bring it up to shoulder level. Gradually, the raised hand will become a signal for the dog to be given a treat. The trainer should not allow the dog to come too slow or sluggishly. This exercise should be repeated 10-15 times during a two-hour training session. If the dog doesn't respond to the treat, the trainer will draw attention to his behavior by tying the leash and gently stroking the dog.

The following complications can be introduced when the dog responds to the command "Come", and then runs quickly and interestedly towards the trainer, using a long-distance leash.

* Separate command and gesture control of the dog;
* Training to sit in front the trainer after getting closer.
* a gradual increase in sitting in front of the trainer as it gets closer;
* Calling the dog from any position; training the dog to sit next to the left trainer's feet after being in a sitting position before the trainer.
* Training for success in the presence of distractions
* Control of the dog with or without a leash
* Calling the dog in various positions by the trainer: standing, sitting or lying down, motion from behind a cover, etc.

The trainer should not use any unpleasant or mechanical stimuli when calling the dog. Treating and petting a dog is the best way to get him to come.

When the dog is unable to follow a command or gesture at the trainer in difficult situations, and the distance exceeds 30 meters, the dog quickly runs up the trainer's arm and then sits down.

Potential errors by the trainer and their results

1. 1.

2. After the dog has been brought to the trainer, use painful or unpleasant stimuli.

3. The dog is called in a systematic manner by the trainer, whether it is standing, sitting or lying down. This stops the dog from settling in one of these positions.

Command "Heel".

For a walk, training, or on service, the dog must be able to move near the trainer. It also discipline the dog and trains it to pay attention to the trainer.

The command is "Heel" with a gesture of slapping the left hand on your thighbone.

Reinforcement: stroking, jerking, leash, and lashing.

From the very beginning of training, the movement is applied. Contrast the basic training method.

The initial exercises are done on a flat surface and in simpler conditions. The trainer attaches a short leash to his dog's collar and wraps its free end around his right arm. The trainer then holds the leash in his left hand, at a distance between 20-25 cm and the collar. He takes the mid-leash in his right hand. After initiating the movement, the trainer gives the command "Heel" which causes the leash to jerk along the dog's body for 0.5-2 seconds.

The trainer should start by walking the dog in a slow, controlled manner. This will allow the dog to become more comfortable with the trainer. Once the dog is properly positioned, close to the left foot of its trainer, the last encouragement will be given by the treat, stroking. Each command "Heel", which drowns the dog's conditional reflex, is accompanied with a jerk on the leash. If the dog's running speed is not more than half that of the trainer, it is considered correct.

In the event of turnings or stops, the command "Heel", which is mandatory, is used. If necessary, the leash can be jerked to support the command. When training fast-paced, strong dogs, a strict collar is preferred. If the dog obeys the command "Heel", the dog will move along with the trainer's left foot, and not pull on the leash. In the future, these complications will be implemented:

* Training the dog to be close to the trainer at different speeds of movement

* Training action using the gesture

* Separate command and gesture control of the dog;

* Training for non-failure in the presence of various distractions (animals and people, birds, vehicles, etc.); training for movement close to the trainer without a leash.

This is how the exercise for the conditional reflex through the gesture is done. The trainer holds the leash in his left hand and uses the gesture to free his left hand. After 1-2 seconds, he gives the command "Heel" then jerks the leash. The command and the jerk can be used to support this gesture, but it must not become a conditional stimulus. In the future, the trainer will only use the jerk by the leash.

You can consolidate your skill by correctly executing the command or gesture, as well as reinforce it with a treat, stroking, or unacted command.

Command "Walk"

In any situation, the ability to change into the "stand-at-ease" position is essential. This skill can be used in training, working or any other situations when the dog requires rest. Gesture: To point the right (or left) hand in the direction of the dog's movement.

Application markers -- signs of fatigue in nervous, muscular, and other systems that activate the reflex to freedom. This command is learned from the beginning of training. It is to be practiced throughout the training course. Verbal commands and gestures are used to train the reflex. This is how the exercise should be done. The trainer holds the dog's side and pulls the leash towards his collar. The trainer gives the dog the command to walk.

He should then run fast, running for 15-30 feet while continuing the walk command. After 2-3 seconds, the hand is directed away (gesture), and is then placed on the hip. The trainer allows the dog to run on the leash after the short walk. He calls the dog again after 1-2 minutes, treats it and then repeats the exercise.

The following rules must be followed when performing the exercise: the initial walking should be done on a long leash. Loud commands and abrupt snapping should not be used. While walking, the dog should always be within sight of the trainer. The following complications can gradually be introduced:

* Control of the dog discreetly by command or gesture
* Walking with the following steps:
* Passing the dog to the stand at-ease from any position, including sitting, standing, or being down. •
* Walking close to different stimuli and accounting for the dog's behavior;
* Alternate walking in both the absence and presence of stimuli. Walking unassisted should be avoided.
* Improvement of walking in a zigzag pattern upon command or gesture

This skill is considered perfected when the canine moves quickly in the direction of the walk command or in gesture.

Possible mistakes by the trainer and other consequences

1. A chokechain is used to provide stand-at-ease for the dog. The leash should be short.
2. To give commands with an excessively high tone and leash snatching while walking

3. Stamina development is hindered by frequent standing-at-ease in sitting, lying down, and remaining.

4. Dogs who are unable to walk on leashes can become disruptive and lose their ability to be disciplined.

Chapter 5: Bringing Your Puppy home For the First Time

Dogs can become our best friends. Being a dog owner is one of life's greatest experiences. Puppies are adorable. Many people also admire their loyalty, friendship and obedience. Puppies are loved by both children and their elders. A friendly dog can help you create the perfect family. Although it might seem difficult to begin a new life with a puppy, with training and passion you can make your dog a valued member of the family.

How do you bring your puppy home?

You should make sure you are ready for your puppy. It is a big step to add a new member of your family. You must take care of the emotional side. Animals have different needs. Separation anxiety can really hurt your relationship with your puppy. Your puppy will have his own desires. Don't let your puppy feel alone. You can be a good partner. You will need to know some rules in order to do this. Rules are not just for dogs. You will need to adapt to the dog's different habits and routines as the adult.

The first time you bring a puppy home

It's exciting to bring a puppy home. Everyone is discussing their desire to adopt a puppy, and the habits of their dog. How do you announce your puppy's arrival into the family? What's the best gift you can give your puppy as a start? Be aware that every puppy comes with some sleepless nights. Prepare for it. To make your dog a friend, it will take patience and time.

Tips for the first time

Your puppy will be most comfortable being called by his name when he arrives at your house. He will soon learn to recognize his name. Because the puppy is separated from his family, he may feel lonely and upset at first. The puppy should be calm for the first week. Let the animal explore his new home and get to know the family members. You should ensure that your puppy relieves himself in the designated area. Your puppy should be taken to the designated area. Give him time to relieve himself. Be quiet if he doesn't do it in the right place. When he does it, praise him.

You should never let your puppy out of sight. Take him with you around the house. Talk to your family about creating a safe environment for your dog. Give your puppy a place where he can feel relaxed.

To make your pet feel secure and safe, you can provide a small crate. You should not let your puppy sleep in your bed. It will be difficult at first, as your puppy may cry all night. He will eventually learn his sleeping habits and place.

The well-being and welfare of Mother Nature is naturally tied to animals. They are naturally inclined to love and give. Your responsibility is to train your puppy. Young puppies don't have consciousness. Remember that puppies and humans are very different. People often treat their dog as if it were a friend. It is possible to train your dog to behave humanely, but it may not work for the best.

The ability to think is given to human beings, which makes us different from animals. Because we can think, we have the ability to choose. We know the difference between good or bad, which is why the religion has the concept of heaven and hell. These things are known because we have the option to choose. Animals don't have the option, as they are unable to think like us. It will be an interesting experience to share your knowledge with them. They can't hear you, but they can feel your presence. They can't read your facial expressions but they can understand your voice. They can listen to your heart and understand your mood. My dog will often sit with me when I'm not feeling well. He wants me not to stress. My dog is a special friend and I feel a strong connection to him. This led me to write this book. Your dog is the best judge of how you should treat him. You only need to be patient with your dog and love him.

Let's get started together.
Why should you train your puppy?
Dog training requires patience and time. People often ask me why I should train my dog. The puppy should be brought home at eight weeks of age. You should not bring your puppy home before she is eight weeks old. Six weeks old. The most important concepts for puppies to master in life are bite inhibition, potty-training, and sleeping. These concepts may not be taught to the puppy until she is eight weeks old. However, the mother will continue basic training. Eight weeks is the ideal time to begin training your puppy. Puppies are more playful at this age. Training begins on the first day.

Dog behavior problems can cause confusion in people. Your puppy is your best friend and you care about his health. The puppy doesn't like you, even though you treat him as a member of your family. You suddenly notice a change in his behavior. He barks at you and ignores you. These types of problems can make people feel helpless. They don't know what to do.

These problems can be traced back to poor training or no training at all, according to my experience.

Your dog doesn't know how to behave with you and your rules. You have the responsibility to teach your dog, and you should treat him as a loving parent. Dog training requires patience and time. It is best to not sleep with your dog for the first four weeks.

Dogs that are not willing to obey commands can be a problem. This is why it is so important to train your dog. These are just a few of the many reasons why you should start puppy training.

Training your puppy is vital for your safety and for your dog's well-being. To have a long-lasting partnership, you must get to know each other.

You will need to train your dog in order for him to live a happy and healthy life. Pets are not happy for humans to interrupt their lives. They don't want to be trained and can't learn the skills by themselves. You can both agree to train them. You should tell them you're going to live together and that you will need to create a shared life.

The puppy will treat your house like his bathroom if he is not properly trained. Because the puppy doesn't know how to relieve himself, you will not be able live in your home. Find a place for the puppy to relieve himself. To live a happy life, you must provide good training.

Be consistent throughout the training. Your commands will gradually be understood by the dog. To help your dog learn about your instructions, it will take a long training period.

Training will make it easier to show your puppy off to your friends. Your puppy will be awkward if you don't train him.

Without good training, you can't participate in pet competitions. People show their dogs at these training sessions. You will feel embarrassed in front of others if your dog is not obeying commands.

Your dog's safety is guaranteed by training it. For a long-term commitment, it is crucial that your dog trusts you and your associates.

Training requires patience

Humans appeared on Earth 2.5 million years ago, according to history. Humans have amazing abilities thanks to their long evolutionary processes. Humans are distinguished from other animals by their ability to think and distinguish. Intelligence and wisdom are gifts that humans have been given. We believe we are intelligent. We are capable of running large industries and making big decisions. You know what? Humans make stupid mistakes. This was something that took me a while to grasp.

If your dog is not able to sit, all the years of practice are meaningless. Dog training is no different. It took 2.5 million years for us to get here. It will take patience and time. I will repeat it: Dog training takes time, patience, and time. I do not like repetition. However, I have found that persistence is the best way to succeed.

It is important to have compassion, empathy, compassion, love, and respect for all animals. According to "Our ultimate reality", animals are better than humans because they have a better quality of life. While I don't want to create a conflict between pets and people, I will say this: Never use your power. Do not look down on your pets. Positive reinforcement techniques can be used to help your dog.

Positive reinforcement is rewarding your dog for doing a good deed. Positive reinforcement does not involve punishment or evoking fear. You can give the reward away if the behavior is unacceptable. This section will teach your dog patience. Let's go on this journey together, and then let's move onto the practical steps.

How to teach your puppy to sit and stay

After the puppy has explored your home, training sessions should begin immediately. To make sure your puppy knows his name, call him with the name of your dog. Your puppy will soon remember its name within a few days. You can begin training your puppy as soon as it is eight weeks old if you do so within 1-2 days of its arrival.

You can take your dog to a beautiful place outside. It should be on your lawn, in the garden, or at a park nearby. Let's start with the most fundamental commands: sit, stay, and lay down.

Sit

Bring your dog to the park. The leash should be kept on your knees to ensure that your dog doesn't wander off. You can reward the dog with a treat in your hand. Your hand should be held high above the dog's head. Don't let go of the reward. Guide him to sit when he is paying full attention to your reward. Encourage him to sit. Use a polite and positive tone to tell him "SIT." If he listens attentively while sitting down, praise him immediately and reward him.

Lie Down

Bring the puppy to the exact same spot. Place the puppy in a sitting position. Give him the reward. To grab his attention, show him the reward. Slowly lower your hand to the ground. Your dog will follow you hand. Make him lie down. In a positive tone, tell him to lie down.

Stay

This command has been the most effective in my experience. This command teaches the dog patience and obedience. Let's get started.

Your dog should be allowed to sit in the same position. Give the reward to your dog. Now, let him wait. Move a little closer to your dog, then open your hand and give the reward. You will now speak "STAY" and praise the dog for his good behavior.

This is a checklist to help you train your dog. This checklist contains some basic tips that you should follow. In two days, most people forget the basic rules of puppy training. This can cause serious problems.

Get started as soon as you can.

Clearly speak the name.

To give instructions, use the same voice tone every time. Dogs cannot comprehend the words. They only understand the tone and frequency of the voice. You must make sure that he understands the instructions.

The puppy may be hungry or lonely so start training him. This is the best time for you to reward him.

Do not beat or tease your dog. This can cause him to become anxious and have a negative effect on his emotional and physical well-being.

Positive reinforcement is a way to teach commands.

Rewards can include food or a tennis ball.

Do not teach if you are angry, frustrated, or tense. Do not associate training with negative environments.

So that you are happy and can feel appreciation for your new family member, keep the training sessions brief. Training sessions can be held 2-3 times per day. You should train often. Although you might feel tired after several sessions, it will be worth it when your dog responds correctly. You and your puppy will soon become close friends within a few weeks.

Train your dog to walk on the lead

It is crucial to receive this training. I've met many people. There are no easy rules to training your dog. Leash training can be started immediately or delayed. For puppies under three months old, you can start with a simple flat collar. After a while, you can change to a different collar. You don't want to make your puppy fearful so attach the collar only when he is happy. To gain his trust, you will need to make him feel safe with you. Be patient and take your time. Allow your puppy to take as much time as he needs in order to learn about the world around him.

Slowly attach the leash, showing your affection. Give him a treat, such as a toy, or a food item. Give him the reward, and he will respond. Slowly let go and throw the ball some distance. Let the dog run free on the leash. Show him the food and then ask him to come to your side. You will find that he won't move the first time, so be patient. Let him know that you are rewarding him and let them come to you. Give him the reward when he comes to you.

Chapter 6: Why is Dog Training Important?

Dog training is important for many reasons. It helps you hold your dog responsible for his actions. It's not a good idea to have your dog pouting on people or the mailman, especially if he has your daily mail.

You have control

Your dog shouldn't be taking you on a walk or dragging you along the streets. He should be walking alongside you at the pace that is set by you. Dogs should be able to interact with people and other animals.

You can do less cleaning

Potty training is important because it prevents you from spending hours cleaning up mess in your home. It's a good idea for your dog to go outside to the bathroom.

There is less frustration

Dog training teaches your dog who is boss. Dog training teaches your dog who is in charge. It is your responsibility to run the house, not your dog. It will not get better if you don't have control of the situation.

Your relationship with your dog may be strained. If you take your dog with you, you may feel anxious. You don't want other people to feel anxious around your dog.

Many dogs are left behind because their owners have given up on them. As the dog grew older, they couldn't deal with the bad behavior. The dog is responsible for the bad behavior, but not the owner. It is possible that the dog became aggressive due to confusion about how to behave.

These methods will help you train your dog. They won't happen overnight but they will improve enough to encourage you to keep using the methods you already have.

Lower Injury Risk

The risk of injury is higher when your dog doesn't know how to behave. His actions can cause injury to you or others. Your dog's actions can cause injury to you or others. For example, your dog might jump on someone and knock them over.

The Natural Instincts of Change

It is important that you remember that dogs are naturally instinctive. They may be treated as family members, just like we treat humans. They are an entirely different species than us. You are encouraging a dog to develop natural instincts when you train it.

Because it is his nature to please his owner, he will work hard to change those behaviors. Positive reinforcement is crucial. In a future chapter, we will discuss this.

Reduce aggressive behavior

We can be confident that our dog will protect us from any kind of harm, but we don't want him being aggressive on a daily basis. Many people are unaware that aggression is not about dominance.

It is about managing the situations around him. It's about anxiety and confusion. Fear or frustration can cause it. Until you teach your dog, your dog won't be able to know how you want him to behave in certain situations.

Find out His Needs

Although behavior training a dog is meant to foster a relationship, it is important to consider his needs. Dogs need food, shelter, play and companionship.

Your training efforts must be put in place to ensure he has a happy and safe life. It is important to research the needs of the breed of dog that you own. These can differ depending on:

Age

Breed

Gender

Spayed/neutered, or not

Mental stimulation

Your dog will benefit from the mental stimulation that you provide by training him. This will help your dog to be more alert, happy, and reduce stress and anxiety. Dogs can have many of the same mental issues as adults, which is something most people don't realize.

Dogs that aren't given enough exercise or attention can become depressed. Dogs who are kept chained up for too long may become more aggressive and stop eating.

It is now that you are aware of the importance of dog training, it is time for you to get started. You can't do everything at once with your dog. Only make one or two small changes at a given time. You can introduce more elements once your dog is comfortable with them.

Chapter 7: Get to Know Your Dog

You may be surprised at the differences between a puppy and a dog in adulthood if you've never owned one. You may be surprised to find out that many dogs as young as two months old still behave like a puppy. To ensure your dog is happy and healthy, it's important to understand the different stages of life. The life stage of your dog will also affect the training techniques you use. Young dogs are more receptive to training and may need simpler or less complicated techniques. This chapter will discuss the characteristics and differences between the three stages in a dog's lifespan: puppyhood, adulthood and seniorhood.

Puppyhood

We all know that puppies can be so adorable. It is amazing to watch them grow up before your eyes. It is a wonderful experience to see your dog learn, grow and develop new skills. They can be very demanding, exhausting, and persistent. People who adopt a puppy must be patient during the first few months.

Puppy learning begins immediately at birth. Between 2 and 4 months of age, puppies are most open to learning. As we have already mentioned, this is the best time to socialize your puppy to avoid fearfulness and skittishness in the future. Responsible dog owners must socialize their puppy from this age and start house training.

Puppies need a lot of care, especially in the first few weeks after they arrive. Younger puppies excrete more often so it is important to take them outside frequently to help them learn to use the potty. They should be able to control their bladder and should eliminate between 5 and 8 times per day after the first few weeks.

You should ensure that your puppy is being fed high-quality puppy food with all the required nutrients. Human food can cause problems in the growth of your puppy's bones, muscles, and other organs.

From the time puppies are three months old they need to be fed four meals per day. After that, you can feed them three meals per day.

Another characteristic of puppies is their tendency to chew in a destructive way. Chewing strengthens teeth and provides mental stimulation in the dog world. It's a puppy way to learn about the world and their environment. To prevent your dog from ruining your shoes, give them plenty of chew toys. It is also a good idea to teach your puppy what toys are appropriate for chewing on.

Adulthood/Adolescence

You might be thinking that the joy of puppyhood is over. Dogs can experience the same challenges as humans during their adolescence. Dogs also experience puberty. This is when they undergo a series hormonal changes. Between the ages 6 and 18 months, dogs reach adolescence. Your dog may experience mild pain during this period due to their growth spurts. Your dog will need a lot of chew toys during this time to ease the pressure on their jaws. This is also when their baby hair begins to fall and their adult hair starts growing in. This will lead to more hair loss.

Between the eighth and the twelfth months of their adolescence, dogs reach sexual maturity. The majority of sexual maturity symptoms can be alleviated by spaying or neutering your dog prior to this time. This will prevent them from having their first heat. Your female dog may be more excited to play with other male dogs. If your dog hasn't been spayed by this point, it is important to supervise them when they are out and about. You may not be aware that they might get pregnant. Female dogs need to urinate more often as they grow up. Female dogs may also develop aggressive behaviors towards other female dogs. To prevent undesirable behaviors and actions, make sure that you continue to reinforce and train your dog's good behavior.

Adolescent dogs may also show aggressive behavior. Their bodies produce more testosterone, which leads to more extreme behavior. Male dogs begin to hold other dogs accountable for their duties based on the dog's social hierarchy. This can lead to fights with other dogs. Male dogs need to be taught these feelings and responsibilities. This takes patience and training. Marking is another common problem among adolescent male dog breeds. You can prevent this by having your dog neutered before puberty, or with the proper training.

Boredom and anxiety are likely to be the cause of your adolescent's destructive behavior. To prevent destructive behavior, make sure your dog does lots of exercise. To be calmer at home, they need lots of mental stimulation. Training your dog during their adolescence can be a great time. They are still learning about people and animals. Your dog will be able to tell the difference between people they know and those they don't. Be patient with your dog as you go through this crucial stage of life.

Seniorhood

Did you know that dogs who are older tend to be happier? Because they are used to their routines and have the ability to give all of their attention and affection, older dogs tend to be happier. Different breeds will reach seniorhood at different points in their lives, just like adolescence. However, it is important to be aware of when your dog will reach this age. This could mean that they need to make changes to their diet, exercise, nutrition, and overall health. Your veterinarian will be able tell you when your dog should start making changes.

Voicive some common issues in senior dogs:

Hip dysplasia is a condition that makes it difficult for dogs to run or walk. Depending on the severity of the condition, medication or surgery may be an option.

Orthopedic problems are a condition that results from normal wear and tear of the bones and joints in your dog's body. This stage of life is where arthritis is most common in dogs.

Hypothyroidism is a condition that slows down your dog's metabolism and can lead to obesity or heart disease. This condition can be easily diagnosed with a simple blood test, and managed with medication.

Eye problems: Older dogs can develop eye conditions such as cataracts or hamper vision, which can lead to blindness.

Cancer: This is a common condition that can affect any age of a dog, but it is more prevalent in older dogs.

Dogs can experience confusion as they age and memory problems. Due to declining kidney and bladder function, they may have to use the toilet more often. There is a greater chance of cancers or infections in the reproductive organs if your dog has never been spayed or neutered. You can spot signs early by keeping an eye on your dog. Some of these issues can be treated with medication. These times are important for your dog. Don't force any changes. To prevent injury, pain, or further deterioration, you should avoid jumping and vigorous running.

Your dog may become more independent as he/she gets older. Talk to your vet about the resources that you have to make your dog's life easier. To help your dog live a normal life, you can make small adjustments to your home. This is the most important time in your dog's life.

There are differences between dog training and puppy training

Most people have heard the expression, "You can't teach an older dog new tricks." However, this is not true. It is not easy to teach an older dog new tricks. However, the truth is that it can be difficult. Reinforcement is the most important thing in training a dog, regardless of its age or previous life experiences. It doesn't matter how many tricks you teach your puppy, if you don't reinforce it often enough, they will quickly forget them all. We'll be discussing how age and past experience influence a dog's training, as well as the differences between training a puppy and a dog.

How age and life experience influence a dog's training

You have already learned about the main differences between the three stages in a dog's life: puppyhood, adulthood and seniorhood. These differences make it clear that different training methods will be required for each stage. While the techniques are similar, the methods you use to teach them will differ.

You can teach puppies more quickly than you can with adult dogs. Puppies are more impressionable than adult dogs. They are also more likely to forget if you don't reinforce their behavior. Adult dogs, especially if adopted, often have a basic knowledge. You don't need to spend as much time socializing them as you would with a puppy. However, you can reinforce the desirable behaviors you find appealing.

If you don't have a complete picture of your adult dog's history or what they know, it's best to start to understand what they know. You should test important behavior things such as:

Do you have a dog that jumps on furniture?

Is your dog allowed to go outside for the toilet?

Do you think your dog knows the basics of commands (sit/stay, down, go, leave it, come),?

Do you think your dog knows more advanced commands such as rollover, play dead and stand?

Is your dog able to walk on a leash without being tethered?

Does your dog jump on people?

Does your dog beg for food?

Knowing what your dog knows will help you to determine what behaviors you wish to teach your adult dog. Adult dogs are less likely to be able to learn new behaviors and cues than puppies. However, adult dogs will be more consistent in their reinforcement. Because puppies are constantly doing a variety of actions, it can be difficult to reinforce the correct behaviors. You should schedule training sessions several times per day if you want to teach your dog a new cue. Consistent training will help your dog learn faster and allow you to discover new behaviors and traits about them. Be gentle with your dog during training. There are many examples of dog punishment and how it is often ineffective. Positive reinforcement is the best way to get dogs to behave. In this instance, punishment would take the form of no reward or praise, or even acknowledgment at all. The book's later chapters will provide more information about positive reinforcement.

Training your senior dog should be avoided if he/she is over 50. Older dogs are capable of learning but they have lower energy levels and a weaker body so training sessions should not be too intense. To avoid any deterioration, it is better to reinforce the good behavior of older dogs. Older dogs are more likely to get into accidents in the house due to their weak bladder and impaired kidney function. Reward your senior dog for using the outside bathroom. You can reinforce your senior dog's good behavior by teaching him basic commands and rewarding him for each successful act. These commands can be very helpful in managing your dog and deterring bad behavior. If your senior dog is anxious or aggressive in a situation, you can command them to sit or down. You can make your senior dog's retirement years more enjoyable by continuing to teach them the basics.

There are fundamental differences between training a dog and a puppy

You will need to decide whether you want to train a senior or puppy dog when adopting one. There are many differences between the options. Let's look at some of the most important ones that are related to training.

Puppies can be more work than adult dogs. Puppies must be taught from the beginning how to behave and what not to do. They also need to have a lot of socialization with animals and other people so they don't become fearful and skittish as adults. He/she will learn new things, make mistakes, and have many accidents as he/she matures. Many people are shocked at the amount of work that a puppy requires.

* Adult dogs are more predictable than puppies in terms of size and health. Adopted puppies from shelters are more likely to be from less than ideal circumstances. We don't know enough about their parents to be able to determine if they have any pre-existing medical conditions or temperament issues. Hidden conditions in puppies may need special attention or training that their owners aren't aware of.

* Shelter-reared puppies are more likely to have received no vet attention before they arrived. Shelters usually provide medical care, vaccinations and treatment for disease. It is possible that the puppy hasn't had much other than shelter care, so behavioral issues won't be apparent until they move into their new home. To ensure that the puppy is well-trained and comfortable in their new environment, this will require additional training.

* Senior and adult dogs already have emotional maturity. This means there are less chances of aggression and other undesirable behavior problems. Adult dogs

do not need training. This is because they have been exposed to many things and will not need as much training.

* Senior and adult dogs are great pets to start with. Because they are familiar with basic commands and house training, adult dogs don't require as much training. An adult dog is an excellent option if you don't have the time or energy to properly train and socialize your puppy. Instead of training your dog from scratch, reinforce good behavior and curb bad behavior.

* An adult/senior canine companion is a good way to know what you're getting into. You can interact with an adult dog to see what you're getting into. It is possible to see the physical characteristics of the dog and gain a sense of their temperament. Even though shelter dogs don't usually show their true temperament until they have settled into a home, it is still possible to get an idea of where to start in terms of reinforcement and training.

* Senior and adult dogs can be just as affectionate as puppies. You are wrong to

think that senior dogs will not show the same affection as puppies. Dogs are resilient and open-hearted and can overcome their past in just a few days. While some dogs may have more baggage than others; your dog will remain loyal to you for the rest his/her lives if you show love, affection and care.

The above comparisons will help you get a better idea of what you can expect from each dog, whether it is an adult or a puppy. People who aren't able to dedicate the time necessary to training a puppy should not do so. They can be a lot more work than they realize. Many veterinarians and dog trainers advise puppy owners to take several weeks off work in order to properly train their puppy.

Chapter 8: Basics Of Dog Training

You may have noticed that there are many dog training methods that are used to make the owner feel good, rather than doing what is best. Let me show you (this is particularly important when training difficult breeds like beagles).

If you only use the "positive only" method, your dog will only learn to listen to you when food is available.

Let me explain. This is what you refer to as bribery. If your dog does what you want, you give him a reward. But if he doesn't listen, you don't do anything. Nothing happens.

You won't do anything that could hurt your dog's feelings.

You may wonder, "What's the problem with this?" It doesn't work. Ok, this may be a question for many dog owners. But, let me assure you that I am not saying you shouldn't use tricks when training your dog.

You can use treats in certain situations, such as when your dog is learning tricks.

These situations are not crucial, so it doesn't matter if your dog follows your instructions.

You can't risk chaos if your dog doesn't shake hands with anyone. The basics of obedience training should be your main focus.

Imagine you are walking your dog to the park and your dog starts barking at other animals. You don't have any treats for him. How do you spell it? D-I-S -A-S -T-E -R.

This is true if your dog jumps on strangers due to your inability to properly train your beagle. Even if you do have treats with you, sometimes your dog is too focused on the squirrel chaser than your biscuit.

Respect Training Works

Let's now move to the part that lets you give up on positive-only training. We will talk about how respect training can help your beagle become a better dog.

This is where balance comes into play in your dog training. You can reward your dog's actions with positive reinforcement, but there will also be times when you must let your dog suffer the consequences.

Let's face it, your dog is a living being, just like you and I. To learn, any living creature must experience both the good as well as the bad.

There are two things you need to remember:

* Positive outcomes inspire us to take the same action

* We are discouraged from taking action because of negative consequences

Let me paint you a picture to help you understand what I am trying to convey. Imagine that your mom would reward you with ice cream for every perfect score in your exams. This would encourage you to do the same thing again.

Let's now change the scenario. Let's say that you missed a class and your mom discovered. You were given a stern lecture right away. You would avoid this from ever happening.

This is not a problem that only humans have, it can also happen to dogs. Mother dogs can correct their puppy's behavior by instinct. If a puppy is too rough with Momma Dog, Momma Dog will tell her puppy that this behavior is unacceptable.

Even dogs do this to their puppies. If the puppy is playing rationally, his mom will naturally respond positively. If the situation was not the same, the mom dog will immediately growl.

Ask yourself this question: Does your puppy become bored with his mother or stop playing with him?

Yup, the puppy does not stop playing. He actually continues to play but on a more gentle note. This is what I am trying to convey.

Balanced dog training is the best way to teach your Beagles how to be happy. This means that their actions and behaviors can have a positive or detrimental impact on their consequences.

Positive consequences do not necessarily mean that you should only reward your dog with treats. Your beagle can also enjoy a variety of toys, games and even pet care products.

Negative consequences can be addressed by using a correction word, your voice, body language, tone, and hands cues. You may also consider putting your dog on a leash.

Yes, you're wrong if you think negative consequences of being abusive to your dog are related. It is possible to correct bad behavior without causing harm to your beagle.

If your friends and family only use positive-only training, you should be aware. This e-Book will cover more details.

Chapter 9: Understanding your dog's needs is key

Dogs need to be fed and petted. These are just two basic ways to communicate with your pet. When you decide to get a dog, there are many complex aspects to consider. Are you able to understand why your dog acts strangely or barks "without reason?" There are a few tricks that can help you understand why your dog behaves differently. Dogs' behavior is determined by their owner. They are loyal and will adopt the same feelings and temperament as their master. Don't treat your pet like a toy. You can train your dog in no time. All you need to do is establish a strong relationship between you and your pet.

Dogs will sometimes chew on and damage objects in your home or garden for a time. This happens when puppies are young and their dentition changes. They will be irritated by this process and will destroy everything around them to relieve the stress. They are not to blame for this, and violence is not the answer. The problem should resolve itself once the dentition process has finished. Your dog will cease chewing all things. There may be instances where dogs continue to cause havoc in your home or garden. This could be due to a variety of factors. Stress from frequent departures or arrivals of their owners can cause a disruption in their loyalty. Excessive petting while the master is at home can also lead to spoiled dogs.

A lack of authority from the master is another common problem that can cause instability in a dog-owner relationship. This does not mean that you should isolate your dog by placing him in another room. This can lead to a loss of trust and stress for your dog. If the owner comes home to find a damaged object, the best thing for the pet is not to punish or blame it. The punishment will be incongruous and the pet will lose trust.

One reason your dog is acting out in an unruly manner could be boredom or a change to their daily routine or diet.

You should not punish your dog with beatings or harsh punishments. They will not associate their bad behavior with the mistake they made. Instead, they will view it as punishment for not doing anything wrong and they will lose trust in you.

Remember that a good education may also help with the chewing habit. Most people don't look at their dogs when they play with them. It will give them the impression that they are having fun and will not see it as a problem. You and your children should not blame the dog for chewing on their personal items, such as dolls or fluffy balls. This will teach your dog to respect you and not see it as a problem. A punishment for this reason will cause emotional distress to the dogs and confuse their feelings.

How to correct the behavior of your dog

To change your dog and teach him the right way, you must first identify the problem. The second step is to get your dog to trust you. You must also learn how to give authority to your dog.

Once you have resolved the trust issues, it is time to train your animal. You can teach them basic commands like SIT-WAIT and DEEP-WAIT, or you can even walk at your own pace. Training should be done 2-3 times per day in your home at first. When your dog does a good job, give them a treat. Once you have achieved a satisfactory result, it is time to take your dog outside and begin practicing the same training. It is essential because the dog will perceive outside and inside worlds differently and will act differently if this is not done. Each week, the dog should be taken to another area to explore. You should keep your dog on a leash of five meters. Don't over-pray it. Reward it for coming at you. This is a sign that your training is working. This exercise should last between 20 and 30 minutes.

If the dog is left alone, he should be given a treat. This will encourage him to chew the bone and reduce the stress of being alone. This will make them feel valued and appreciated. If your dog chews on an object near you, call him or her by name to give them a bone. You can distract the dog and reward him with a bone.

It is best to ignore your dog for five seconds before you leave the house. This will reduce the emotion of separation and make your dog feel less sad. Psychologically, this will make your pet more resistant to separation.

The dog should not be allowed to go outside until you return home. You can begin to show affection and care once your pet is able to relax, sit or fall asleep. You should not show your love by placing hands near the door. Doing this will encourage your dog to jump on you and any other people who enter your home. The door is the part that your dog associates with departure and arrival. This is the hardest part. It is the gateway between being seen and being alone. You should not show your dog affection at home, even though it may be difficult. Your dog will feel the joy and excitement from you. You should ignore this radiant joy until you are able to reward your dog with warm or cold petting.

Do not punish your dog if it destroys an object. Your dog will not understand why you are there and may feel guilty for doing so. You don't have to punish your dog for causing damage in a room. Just ignore the problem and wait for the animal to leave the area. You can then clean up the mess.

You should restrict your dog's access to other rooms when you are away. Your dog should be kept in a small, comfortable room with food and toys, but not too many, depending on how long you are away. You should also use this space for your dog when you're home. Otherwise, the dog will be confused and think it is being punished.

Chapter 10: How do you train your dog?

Dogs might be man's best friend, but that doesn't mean they are instinctive like ours. Or that they will adapt naturally to human social environments and not needing any assistance.

You must spend more time with your dog to build a good relationship.

Why should you train your dog?

People who love dogs the most tend to believe that dogs are loyal, committed animals that can understand human emotions and can act as well as humans. Problem is, in the above sentence, dogs are just animals.

Dogs will behave like other animals if they are not trained. Keep in mind that dogs were domesticated wild animals approximately 10,000 years ago. This was just in time to witness the Agricultural Revolution. Some experts believe that domestication began between 30,000 and 100,000 years ago.

According to the US Center for Disease Control and Prevention[1], an estimated 4.5 million Americans are bitten by dogs annually,

Half of these children are children. One in five needed medical attention. In 2012, approximately 27,000 were bitten and required reconstructive surgery. People who live in homes with dogs have a higher chance of getting bitten.

If you are a dog owner and prefer to live with your dog, remember that your dog will behave the same way in the wild as it does in training.

There are many reasons to train your dog. Here are the top five.

Your life and that of your dog will be better. Imagine living with a dog who doesn't respect your home rules or your privacy every day. Your favorite leather chair will be torn or your kitchen floor strewn with dog poop.

Your dog will become responsible and well-mannered by the training you give her. Your dog will be happy if you are well-mannered. Dogs' minds are like children at two years old. He will be more comfortable with being praised for his good deeds than being scolded for his bad ones.

Your dog's safety and that of your family members will be improved by training her. While training your dog to show off is great and fun, it can also save your life.

It is equally important to train your dog well so that you promote safety for all members of your family.

Your dog's instincts are natural and it won't be able stop them, especially if it is not trained well.

Your dog will benefit from mental stimulation when you train her. While it is important to ensure your dog is getting enough physical activity every day, it is equally important that you give her regular mental stimulation through training.

Dogs can be competitive. Your dog can be very competitive. She gets satisfaction from learning or completing a routine. She will also be happy if you give her treats if she is able to learn a new trick or perform a routine.

Dogs are social animals. Dogs prefer to live with other dogs, even in the wild. As a dog owner, you must make your dog feel secure that you are the pack leader. Communicating with your dog regularly is one of the best ways to do this.

Your dog may not speak English as its mother tongue. Training opens up communication channels between you and your dog. This allows you to communicate with your dog in a clear way.

Happy dogs are made of well-mannered, trained dogs. Dogs that are well trained and behaved can get more freedom, or even simple responsibilities. Dogs who are trained can go free and roam the house without being tied down. A well-mannered dog will be loved more and get more praises from people, even strangers. This makes the dog happier.

Training your dog is an important part of being a responsible guardian.

To prevent potential tragedies that could involve your dog, or others, and to help her live a happier and more fulfilled life, you should train her to control her animal instincts.

Positive reinforcement is a great way to build a stronger, more fulfilling, and long-lasting relationship with your dog.

Preparing for the learning environment

You are now responsible for training your dog once you have decided to be a dog owner. It is important to plan what you will teach your dog. You must prepare your dog and yourself, but you also need to create a learning environment.

Here are some ways to make your home conducive for training your dog.

Learn more. You can learn more about dogs and their behavior, as well as how to train them.

You can dog-proof your home. You can avoid frustrating situations such as finding out that your dog destroyed your home or damaged your garden. Sometimes, it is best to prevent such situations from ever happening.

Keep garbage and other items dogs find attractive out of reach.

You should create a place for your dog to express its wild, animal instincts. If necessary, redecorate your home and create a special space for your dog.

This can be a great place to take your dog if you don't have much space at home. Make it a point that your dog knows that the park is the only place it can run and jump freely.

You can make this space as small as a corner of your living room, where you keep your dog's toys. This is a good idea if you don't want your dog getting used to chewing on leather sofas.

Chapter 11: The Basic Commands

Sit

There are many ways to teach your dog how to sit. First, you can capture your dog. Simply, you will be standing in front your dog and holding a treat. You will need to wait for your puppy to sit down before you can give them the treat. Next, encourage them to stand. Wait for them to get up again before giving another treat. Continue this process several times and encourage them to sit.

Luring is the second trick. You can lure your dog by placing a treat in front of them. Just place the treat on their noses and gently lift it above their heads. They can then sit up and reach for the treat by lifting their heads. When their bottom touches the ground, give them the treat. Continue this process several times, then reward them with an empty hand.

This will enable them to understand the hand signal and associate the command with "sit".

However, it is best to not physically sit your dog. This could cause them to become confused or upset.

Down

This is another command that you need to teach your dog. Be sure to not confuse them by saying "down" while you are telling them to get up from the couch.

Simply hold a treat in your hands and let a small amount of it stick out. This will train them to go lower. Your pup will be able to see the treat. Then, show it to your pup and place a treat underneath in a flat hand. They will be able to reach it as many times as possible. Give it to them once they are comfortable and relaxed.

Continue repeating this until they understand that their hands are on the ground and they must lie down. Make sure you include the verbal cue "down", so they can follow your lead every time you say it. They will eventually learn to lie down when they are asked, even if you don't give them a treat.

Stay

If your dog understands the verbal cue "stay", they will likely remain still until you ask them to stand or give you a release cue. Staying in place is a behavior that can be sustained. This is a way to get your dog to sit still until you give a cue.

First, choose the release word you want to use.

Begin by sitting or standing with your dog. Next, place a treat on the ground and let them reach for it. Repeat this process several times until your pup understands that the release cue is to get up and move to your feet.

Reward your furry friend for mastering the sit and release cues. Give them another treat if they remain in the sitting position as you ask. Slowly increase the amount of time between treats so they can wait longer for the release cue. It is okay if they get up and leave the room without the release cue. This simply means they aren't ready to sit for prolonged periods of time.

After they have mastered the ability to sit for a few seconds, increase their distance. Then ask them to sit down and remain there for a few seconds. Next, take a moment to step back and let them rest. Give them a treat, and then let them go. You can keep building up, making it easier for them to stay put until they release you. This can be done facing them or when you are walking away with your back to them.

However, you shouldn't expect too much of your dog. It is important to remember that training goals can only be achieved in small steps. Therefore, it is important to have patience and take each step one at a time. Remember to keep sessions short and effective.

Walking on a loose leash

The command "heel", which is used to train your dog in obedience, means that your dog should be walking on your left side and their head aligned with the knee of your hand as you loosely pull the leash. Your friend will be able to walk more politely if you let the leach go without pulling. Others prefer to use the words

"let's go" and "Forward" for easy walking with their dog.
Which cue do YOU prefer?
It doesn't matter what you like, but it is important that you stick to it. It doesn't matter if your dog walks on your right or left side. That is up to you. It is important that you keep your dog in the same place you want it to so they don't wander off-track.
First, ensure your pet is comfortable with a leash. They might initially feel odd and may bite the leash.

Reward them for every time they put the leash around their neck. Hold the leash loosely on your neck and give them treats for sitting or standing next to you. Encourage them to take a step forward and then give them a treat when they do.
Slowly increase the amount of leash time until your faithful friend is comfortable walking by your side. Allow them to take in

the scenery as you go, and then give them the signal "let's go!" with a happy, appreciative tone. Reward them for returning to their original position and for continuing the walk with your.

Come

This command is important if you want your dog to respond to commands, especially indoors or in quiet areas. Simply sit down with your dog and say "come." You can also say their name to let them know you are there. Give them a treat when you give the cue and they respond accordingly.

Simply drop a treat right in front of them and when they're done, you can say their name again. Give them another treat when they look up. Continue doing this until they are familiar with what to do when you call them. Next, move away from them and start to do it from a distance. Give them a treat when they come running towards you.

It is vital to not say their name too often, as they may ignore you. It is best to get closer to your dog and then move back to call them. They will respond well if you do this. When they are able to turn their heads to face you, you can gradually increase the distance. You can make it more exciting by calling their name and running to chase them. Give them a treat when they catch up to you.

Continue to increase your distances and play at new locations. Do not grab your pet when they approach you. This can be confusing or frightening. If your dog seems timid or afraid, you can kneel down and offer a treat.

Do not call your dog to punish him. They might be trained to associate punishment with the call. Reward them for responding well to your name, even if they are being mischievous.

Chapter 12: Starting Your Puppy off On The Right Paw

Many people wonder when or how old they should train their puppy. Cesar Milan, a famous dog trainer, suggests you get started right away. The sooner you start, the better. These are some tips to help you train and keep your dog obedient from the beginning.

Instead of worrying about the toys and beds you will get for your puppy, you can spend some time thinking about what you want to do with your puppy. A strong leader is an essential biological requirement for your puppy.

Be a strong pack leader. Your dog is wired to follow you as a pack leader. You must have strong, consistent, and stable traits to be a strong pack leader. People who are strong leaders at work may be able to bond with their dogs, but they don't get along well at home. Many people are left to wonder why their dogs behave badly.

Your puppy will sense if you are not confident and try to control you. Bad behaviors like pulling on the leash, chewing up objects, and anxiety can occur when this happens. To ensure your puppy is well-adjusted and balanced, you must show leadership from the beginning. You must be the pack leader for your puppy throughout the training period. It is crucial to keep your role as pack leader for your dog.

Housebreaking. Housebreaking is something that most dogs can pick up easily by the time they are 3-4 months old. Your puppy should be taken outside to the exact same place you want them to relieve their bladders. In no time, they will be familiar with the area and feel at ease. This will allow your puppy to relieve himself regularly.

Be consistent by taking your dog to the place you prefer for them to relieve themselves. It will help them learn the habit. Make sure your puppy gets rewarded for removing themselves from the correct area. You can reward your puppy verbally or with a physical treat. Your dog will be delighted to hear your glowing praises. Your words of praise can help to restore your dog's mental stability.

Dog Walking. Your puppy's pack leader should find creative ways to give them energy and the exercise they need. Dog owners should take their dogs for a walk every day. This will help you be seen as the pack leader by walking alongside your dog. You should always be the first to leave the house and the last to enter the room when you go for a walk. Your dog should always be beside or behind you during a walk.

Seek out a vet. Regular visits to the vet are an important part of maintaining a healthy puppy. Regular exercise and a healthy diet will keep your puppy happy and healthy. Discuss with your vet when is the best time for your dog to be spayed or neutered.

Before you start an exercise program, it is a good idea for your pet to speak to your veterinarian about long-term bone issues, parvovirus, or other health concerns.

Chapter 13: Puppy Training For New Dog Owners

Congratulations to anyone who is thinking of getting a puppy, or to those already with one. This will be a wonderful journey that will bring you to a happy and fulfilling relationship. This guide will not address the benefits or drawbacks of specific breeds. It is important to note and point out that the myth of 'the perfect dog" is false and should be avoided. Here's why:

Every breed of dog has its merits and detractors. Each dog breed also has its unique behavioral and physical characteristics, such as exercise requirements and shedding, and inherent behaviors. These are important considerations if you're not yet ready to buy a puppy. Your lifestyle and other factors will also play a role in choosing the right puppy.

You can research different breeds of dogs to find the one that suits your needs. This is an essential step, and you and your puppy will suffer if it's not done correctly.

You should also consider where your dog will be purchased if it is your first purchase of a puppy or rescue. You should aim to adopt or purchase the pet from a trusted person or organization.

The age of your puppy is another important thing to consider. Your puppy should be between 2 1/2 and 3 months old when you bring him or her home. Here's why. A puppy's first three months of life is crucial. This is when a puppy develops social skills with its mother and littermates. This is the time when the puppy learns to accept discipline and how to respond. It's also where they can begin to understand basic canine body language responses. It's very likely that a puppy less than this age will bite and continue to behave like this throughout adulthood.

You must prepare for your pup before you bring him home. Let's take a look at what you can do to prepare your puppy.

How to prepare for your pet

You need to be prepared before you rush to your car to drive to your purchase location and bring home your perfect pup. You can think of it as preparing for a friend you'll be welcoming into your home within the next week. This applies to you as well. Prepare for your puppy's arrival.

Depending on where you live, the dog breed and other characteristics of your home, preparation will vary. You will need to prepare the equipment necessary for your pup, such as toys, treats and bowls, blankets, blankets, crate, collar, and other items. Preparing for your puppy involves three phases: equipment, house rules and service provider. Let's take a look at the most important part of these phases, equipment. An online search will reveal a variety of house rules that you can modify to your taste.

Preparing the Equipment

The following equipment is necessary to ensure your dog's happiness, comfort, and successful training.

Crate

A crate is the best behavior management tool. The crate prevents your dog from acting out or being disruptive, and allows you to housetrain your dog.

How to choose a crate

Crate training your dog can be a crucial part of raising a happy, well-behaved dog. Many dog owners find it difficult to decide which crate they should buy. These are just a few of the many options. There are five basic types of crates available: wire crates (cute crates), softsided crates (plastic crates), plastic crates (heavy duty crates) and wire crates (5). Each crat has its own advantages and disadvantages. See illustration.

How to Crate Train a Puppy with Separation Anxiety

Your puppy will be sad to go home after the first time. The puppy or dog may appear stressed in this situation. In an attempt to escape, he or she may scratch at walls, chew on walls, bark uncontrollably, scratch at doors or walls, or scratch at them if you are not there. Separation anxiety is when a dog acts and behaves in these ways. Separation anxiety can be a behavioral problem. Separation anxiety is a learned, simulated behavior in which a dog only wants attention when it needs it. This anxiety is caused by a lack leadership and self-control. However, dogs can suffer real stress from being left alone when their master is not there.

Simulated separation anxiety can be dealt with by ensuring that your dog is more comfortable in a crate while you are away than when you are home. This should be accompanied with obedience training, strong leadership, and exercise.

It is important to be kind and loving with your puppy from the moment you bring him or her home. As we have already mentioned, your puppy will be missing his friends and playmates when you bring him or her home. You may feel tempted to touch your dog or take him out of his crate, but this is not the right thing. You are rewarding bad behavior by doing these things.

Instead, you need to teach your dog how to remain calm and peaceful for long periods of time. You should also teach your puppy how to behave calmly, quietly, and patiently. You should also avoid getting too attached to your puppy when training him.

You can control separation anxiety by crate training your dog. When you are at home, crate-train your dog by putting the dog in a crate. Then, gradually increase the time. You can also feed your dog in the crate, and give it a treat or bone. To keep your dog entertained, you can place interactive toys inside the crate.

Notice: Dogs can play with toys
Designed to entertain and
Barking is a common separation anxiety behavior. This behavior can be controlled by teaching your dog the quiet command. A bark collar is also useful if the situation gets out of control.

Note: Crate training your dog will keep him or her from chewing or destroying furniture and footwear. You can also house train your puppy. Referring to house training

How to house train your puppy

House training is the most important thing about house training your puppy.

It is simple to house train a dog. You can housetrain your dog by setting up a schedule for food and allowing the dog to relieve himself or herself outside. Reward the dog when the behavior is successful.

You can eliminate the need to feed your dog every day by setting a routine. The puppy who eats without restriction also eats randomly and freely. It is easier to predict your dog's defecation times if he or she is following a specific feeding schedule. Your dog should go first thing in the morning after breakfast, lunch, dinner, play, and training. When your dog needs to go, you can see it in their behavior. You may see your dog circling, sniffing, and hunching when they need to go. You can train your puppy to recognize these signs as you house-train him or her.

Leash

Another important tool for dog training is the leash. There are many types of leashes. They come in different lengths and sizes. Let's take a look at some of the most common leashes.

Nylon Leashes - Nylon leashes can be found in many places and are often used. Nylon leashes can be purchased in a variety of colors and are both strong and inexpensive. These leashes can be very durable, but they can also cause injury to your hands if your dog is too strong. Because of their lightness, nylon leashes work well for puppies.

Leather Leashes - Leather leashes are loved by many dog owners and lovers. Leather leashes can be strong and last a lifetime. They can be difficult to buy, but they soften as the material ages. Because it is so gentle, this type of leash is great for strong dogs.

Chain Leashes - There are many options for chain leashes. They come in various lengths and prices. The majority of them are inexpensive because they can hurt your hand or cause damage to a dog's teeth.

Cotton Leashes - These leashes are rare. If you plan to take your dog swimming, a cotton leash will be the best choice. However, due to the nature and strength of cotton, you might get rope burns if you use a cotton leash for walking a strong dog. Cotton leashes are great for puppies because of their soft nature.

Leash Length

As long as you have control over your dog, any length of leash is fine. If you plan to take your dog on a walk in a busy area like a city, consider a 4-foot leash. A 6-foot leash is recommended for those who live in suburbs. A leash that is at least 6 feet long is the best for walking your dog in traffic and on busy streets.

How to teach your puppy leash skills

It is important to show your dog basic leash skills. It will be easier for your dog or puppy to walk around the neighborhood, park, or other crowded areas if they are taught basic leash skills. Your safety and that of your dog is paramount. Let's take a look at how to teach your puppy that fundamental skill.

Preparation

First, ensure your puppy or dog has a collar. Next, reward your dog with treats and a clicker. A clicker is a way to mark good behavior. Once you have a list of all the things you need, you can decide which side your dog should be walking on. If you have show-dog inspirations you might teach your dog to follow the standard. You don't need to have show-dog inspirations to choose one side. Otherwise, your dog will be unable to cross the street and fall over if you don't. Let's now look at some tips and tricks that you can use when leash training your dog.

How to get your dog to walk without pulling on the leash

These are some tips to get your dog walking without pulling:

You can train your dog to walk on their own. If your dog pulls or lunges forward, you can let it go. Eventually, he/she will stop pulling and will look back at you in wonder, "hmmmm...Why aren't you just following me?" You can reward the dog immediately and praise him/her. This is known as capturing the right behavior.

Step 2 – Repeat the previous steps several times, and reward your dog or pup. Reward and praise your dog every time he or she walks well without pulling. He or she will eventually associate praise and a treat with good walking. Alternate Method - This alternative method is ideal for training dogs and puppies who are submissive. This method involves halting in your tracks (statue) when your dog pulls on the leash. The dog will be forced to look back, and the leash will become looser. Reward and praise the dog immediately and then start walking. This should be repeated each time your dog lunges forwards.

How to teach your dog to walk by your side

It is easier to get your dog walking by your side. These steps will help you teach your dog to walk along your side if he wanders.

Step 1: To start, put a short leash around your dog. You should ensure that your dog's leash is the right length. It shouldn't be too long that it drags you, or too short that it makes it difficult for the dog to move away from you.

From your destination point of walking.

You can lure him or her to your side with treats and praises when they agree. Use a clicker if you have one to mark the behavior. If not, you can use the word "side", or any other word.

Chapter 14: Havanedze training
What to do if your dog has severe anxiety

Havanedze dog owners face a lot of problems, including anxiety and seraration. Uour dog is extremely loyal and wants to go with the owner wherever he goes. Although we would love for our Havanedze to accompany us wherever we go, that is not possible due to the fact that we need to travel to work or other areas where dogs are not permitted.

You can leave them at home and they will be fine. You will find out that your dog has reeded on the carpet or shewed through your favourite rair of Dzhoedz. It is dzometimedz difficult to imagine your sute Havanese becoming a little mondzter at the home. All besaudze they get worried about you leaving them and won't come back.

Dog Seraration Anxietu: The Sources

Anxiety is rooted in their nature as pack animals. This makes them anxious and causes them to agitate and be unruly. They feel a dzendze detashment after their madzter leavesdz, and that makes them dozturbed. Fast, the owner can take certain actions to build on their anxietu and get them more agitated.

If uou pay attention to them before or after uou go, and this is done on a consistent badzidz everyu dau, the rattern they dzet getdz inseminated in their daily routine and their agitation builddz da after day.

Redusing Dog Seraration Anxietu

You astuallu have a greater impact on their agitation then you might realize. You can reduce their anxiety by including certain shangedz into your astiondz.

These are some simple ways to reduce anxiety.

* You can mix it up ur everu dau. If you have a set number uou must complete each dau before uou go, you may want to change it up a bit. You may find that uour Havanedze can dztartdz ur to assist ur

when uou select ur sar keys for indztanse. If this is the case, you might try udzing another arroash to obtain uour keudz next time. Before you leave, make sure to put uour keys in your rosket. A common trigger is to take them for a walk in the morning before they go. If you know you will be leaving them home after walking them, you can take them on a walk before you leave.

* Stay neutral: It is difficult to not give them an affestion before you leave. You will still be there for them when you leave. But, if you leave them, thidz will only increase their anxiety. This is true even if uou are returning home. It is important not to give them too much attention either before or after they return. To lower their anxiety, the best way is to not disassociate the time spent away and the attention they receive. You can resomend that uou pretend that nothing hadz happened before you leave or when uou return, and that uou ignore your dog for 10 minutes before and afterwards. Do not retort or hug your dog during thodze

moments, even if they make sad noises or are having a difficult time sleeping. You are only helping them to reduce their anxiety when they aren't at home.

Begin with shorter periods. If your dog is anxious as soon as you leave, take them out for a while and then go back in. This will reduce their anxiety about when they will return and how long it will take. You can dzlowlu insreadze when uou depart them, dzo it would seem natural to them that they do some bask regardless of whether uou are gone.

You Are Not Being Mean

It may seem like some of the Havanedze dog owners are cruel. You must realize that thidz can reduce their anxiety which in turn will allow them to be calmer, healthier and happier in the long-term.

Anxiety problems in dogs that have been ragging for some time should be addressed immediately. You don't want your Havanese to discover that they have done something wrong. If that happens, you should immediately redzrond and harrendz besaudze them.

LOVABLE SMALL DOGS THAT ARE HALF HAVANEDzE

The Havanedze, a small dog with dzmall markings, is very sategoriedz. They are friendly with other pets and shildren, are non-dzhed, and have no allergies. What more can you ask for? Many hubrid dogdz are made with the Havanedze. Thidz wau can rodzdziblu choose between two breeds.

Dzmall dog breeddz are popular because they are easier to transport, require less care, are more comfortable with their owners, and can be dzit on our lardz. Manu reorle mixed breed dogdz can be saudze they are healthier and live longer. Dedzigner dogs can be very rorular at the moment, so it dzeemdz like everyuone is trying to find their next bedzt breed.

Havanese dogs are a Cuban breed. They were frequently found in the homes of the wealthy during the 18th- and 19th senturiedz. The 1960dz was a time when Cubandz emigrated to the US. They brought their dogs. Havenedze were first bred in America in the 1970s. There are many solordz for Havenedze: white, black, silver, gold and white. They are known for being intelligent and easy to train. Havanese dogs love to be with their reorle. They have dark eyes and long dzilku hairs that are easy to keep clean when they're kert short. They can be alert and watchdogdz but they also bark a lot. They are prone to dzkin donezeadzedz or satarastdz. The Havanedze and other favored dzmall breeddz make a cute, new dog.

Cavanedze also includes a King Charledz Saraniel and rrodusedz, a dog that can idz 12-17 rounds. They can have different looks. Dzome have surlu, short hair while others have long. They are gentle, patient, loving, and easy to train.

A Poovanese or Havapoo includes a Poodle. They look a lot like a Havanese, but with more surlu hair. Sometimes, theu can be found with a short, docked tail similar to the Poodle. They don't need to be dzhed and are easy to train.

The Havadzhire is a Yorkshire Terrier. They are usually a bit taller than their long counterparts and have a medium-long tail. Their soat idz are long and straight, although some have the hair like a Havanedze. Their beards and euebrowdz have a well-defined appearance. This hubrid was very caring for the 10 ueardz. They are great with children but can take some time to get used to different retdz. Udzuallu are 5-13 pounds in weight and have a high-pitched bark. The Havapeke is also known as the Pekingese. They are of Chinedze heritage. This combination udzuallu gives you a 7-14 pound dog. It needs a lot of brushing. They require very little grooming, but they are friendly with people and can be a bit stubborn. They are difficult to house break and can cause eye and breathing problems.

The Havamalt is a Maltedze. The Havamalt is a loyal, affectionate dog, easy to train, and gentle. Thidz hubrid is a more reliable dog than the few others. They don't bark too much and they are always on the lookout for their watch dogdz. The Thidz dog doesn't doedznt udzuallu dahed, but this is not true for everyone. They become betw12 rounddz.

Anu of the breeddz mentioned above will make a loving, loual family dog. It is important to find a reliable, trudzted breeder or to seek out a redzsue organization that can adopt a needu pet.

HAVANEDzE DOG TRAINING TIPS

Although you may be the biggest dog lover in the world, that doesn't mean everyone in your uour family or sirsle friends is a biggie. Even cute Havanese mau love canines. You might have been a bad dog owner or a child with a dog.

It'dz also possible for them to be scared by the dzresifis behavior your dog may exhibit. It'dz crucial to not only learn about the dog's fear but also to determine what you can do as a dog owner to help it go away.

The Source of Fear

Step 1 idz talk to uour famiilu or frienddz regarding what's going on. Imagine being afraid of the dog'dz owner because it growled at you. What would you think if the dog'dz owners blamed uou because the dog growled at uou?

You shouldn't give the dzame. Alwaudz begin by assuming that there is a sound for their fear. Talk to them about it. Ask them if they have ever seen anything in their dog that could cause fear, or if they were tasked with it as a child. Once you have determined the cause of the fear, uou will be able to begin dealing with it.

If your dog is afraid of you

You should always ask your dog to stop doing something that is causing the problem. Dog owners who are not dog lovers have a tendency to be blinded by the bad behavior of their dogs. Your Havanedze is a beautiful little angel.

You may have a serious rroblem if your friends start to growl when you approach their water bowl. This is not something that can be ignored.

To dztartz with, you must addredzdz your behaviour. If your dog displays aggressive tendensiedz on their territory or space, you should take control and show the dog that you are in charge. Once you've done this, ensure that no one is treating your dog cruelly. Fear breeds in dogs that are irritable, eg if they're on their front or rhudzisal.

If the Fear is from an Insident of the Past

It may be a past event if your dog doesn't seem to be experiencing the same anxiety and fear as your friends or family. It is possible to blame your dog and tell them to "deal" with the situation.

However, would uou really want dzomeone be so insensitive with uou. Probablu not. I am not suggesting that uou hide your dog in a corner until you leave. But, uou should implement security safeguards to ensure your safety at home.

Firdzt, teach uour dog to dztor at dztrangerdz. When new reorle enter your houdze, make sure they are calm and well-behaved. Sesond, let dzure them know that they don't have to greet the dog or pet him.

Most dogdz will ignore you and make it worse. They will all respond in the same way adz thidz, which is a signal that they should be left alone rredzuming it idz not be toushing or sontast.

If uou are patient and well-mannered, uou might be able to show your dog that you don't expect the dog to behave badly. But, it is important to show the dog that you are aware of their behavior.

Chapter 15: Housebreaking Your Puppy in 4 Easy Steps

The boy said, "I'm not alone." "I have a puppy."
Jane Thayer - The Puppy That Wanted a Boy
The key takeaway: Housebreaking your dog helps to establish a happy, healthy relationship. Only after your puppy has been housebroken will you be able to let him roam free.

Housetraining your puppy requires patience, consistency, and lots of positive reinforcement. This exercise is designed to instill good behavior in your puppy and create a loving relationship with it. Your puppy will need to learn how to housetrain in between four and six months. Some puppies may take as long as a year to house-train. It could also be a factor of size.

A smaller puppy will have a smaller bladder and a faster metabolism than a larger pup. A smaller puppy will need to be out more often. You should also consider the living conditions of your pup. You might also need to eliminate undesirable behaviors from your puppy and create desirable ones. It is important to establish a schedule that you stick to.

Be patient

Be consistent and patient. You must remember that you are dealing directly with a puppy. A puppy does not understand English. Your tone and other nonverbal cues are all that a puppy will pick up on. There will be setbacks when you train your puppy. These setbacks shouldn't be a reason to stop training your puppy. Your puppy will be fine as long as you manage them well. If your puppy is showing signs of discomfort, you should immediately take him out. You can reward him for going outside and he will be fine. This will teach him.

How to start housetraining

When the pup is 12-16 weeks old, housetraining can begin. The pup should be able to control his bladder and bowel movements at this age. It will take you longer to housetrain your puppy if he is older than that. It will take longer to housetrain your puppy if he is used to excreting in his cage. Your puppy will be more comfortable being house trained if you reward him with praise and encouragement.

The theory is that housetraining is easier if you limit the space available to your puppy. It will not move from its place of sleep or food. It would therefore want to go outside for its business. These are the steps you should take to housetrain your dog.

Make a schedule

Establish a feeding schedule for your puppy. Between meals, don't let the puppy eat out of his bowl. After a meal, after the pup has had his meal and after play, take the puppy on a walk. After an hour, take him to the bathroom.

Make sure you take your puppy out before he goes back to bed. To make sure your dog can go to his normal spot, you should take him there every time. He will be prompted to do this if he smells it. He will need you to be outside until he's housetrained. When your dog does his business, praise him and give him a treat. You can also give your dog a treat by taking him on a walk.

Use a Crate

A crate is also possible. You should not leave your dog in the crate longer than two hours. You should only allow your dog to sleep in the crate at night. It should be a suitable size. The pup may use it as a bathroom if the crate is too large. It shouldn't be too small for the pup. You will have to be able to spend time with your puppy during the training period. If your puppy uses the crate for elimination, you should get rid of it immediately.

Your puppy should not be sniffing the ground or whining. Potty training is not without its hazards. These incidents will require you to be prepared.

Do not be harsh or irritable with your puppy. Instead, make sure to clean up the area and then take your puppy outside. It will be easier to keep an eye on the puppy and say no when you see it.

Chapter 16: Puppy proofing your house

To keep your dog safe, it is essential that you puppy proof your home. These are some of the things you can do to avoid any injuries.

Living room

Carpets/ Couch

Protect your couches and carpets first. This is especially important for white or cream carpets. It will be soiled by your pooch if he jumps on it. Protective coverings are necessary to keep your pooch safe from falling off any high-rise platform. You should also make sure that you do not place any valuables over these surfaces. Your pooch could jump on it and cause damage. Roll up the carpets until your dog is old enough to unroll them.

Television unit

Protect the edges of a TV cabinet made from wood if you want it to last. Your puppy will likely do the same thing. They chew on wood to strengthen their teeth. These exposed edges can be covered with wood protector strips. It can be covered with cloth strips to prevent your dog from chewing or biting at it.

Sockets

Dogs could be very dangerous around open sockets. To ensure safety, you must cover all exposed sockets. The socket plugs can be used to block them. You should also roll up any wires or cables your dog might chew on. Even if the cables aren't connected, it is possible to connect one that has been chewed on and start a fire.

Stairs

Make sure your dog is safe on stairs and take precautions if it becomes a danger.

Bedroom

Betts

Your pet will be most at home in a bed. They will consider it their home and not their owners'. Puppies won't hesitate to vomit on their beds. Many pets will jump onto the bed right after they eat and end up re-educating their food. Your puppy should not be allowed to sleep on your bed until it is old enough to stop doing this. To prevent your dog from getting into your room, you can lock the doors to your bedroom. If your dog climbs on the bed, you must shout "NO!"

Cupboards / Closets

Your cupboards and closets will be a favorite place for pups to explore. They will chew anything they find rough, so all your expensive clothes are at risk. They will grab anything on a shelf and begin chewing it right away. You can end up paying a lot more than you think. To prevent them accessing your cupboards and closets, lock them.

Shoe racks

Your dog will love to raid your shoe rack and closet. Your dog will not hesitate to rip apart any shoe or slipper. If you have expensive shoes, this can be an issue. Keep your shoes in a closed closet or high up so your dog can't reach them. They will eat socks as well.

Kitchen

Pantry

Keep the pantry locked. Also, make sure there aren't any food packets outside. You can be sure that your dog will not chew anything, even packaged cartons. All your candies and chocolates should be kept in drawers or in a fridge. To prevent your pet's entry, you can keep the kitchen door shut all the time.

Tables

Pets love to chew on the legs of chairs and tables. To sharpen their teeth, they will not hesitate to chew on the legs of chairs and tables. Protecting the legs of these chairs and tables with protective materials such as thick cloths is a good idea. You can keep an eye on them and install cameras all around the house. Spray them with puppy repellant spray to protect your furniture.

Garden

Your pets can find the garden just as dangerous as any other room in the house.

Tools

To keep your pets away from your garden tools, you must lock them all. You can hang them from the garage or place them in plastic containers. You should make sure your pet is safe from sharp objects and implements while they run.

Plants

Certain plants could be hazardous for your pet. They can cause poisoning if they are chewed on. It is important to know the signs and ensure that your pet does not have access to these plants. You might also find thorny plants that could be equally dangerous and injure your pet. These plants can be protected by fencing.

These are just a few of the many ways you can protect your home and prevent injuries to pets.

Chapter 17: How to Teach Your Dog Advanced Skills

Dog Fun Fact: Every dog has its own nose print, just like each human's fingerprint. It is difficult to take nose prints on dogs because their noses are always moist.

Dog Joke: Q. What do you refer to as a large dog who meditates? Aware of the wolf!

Once your dog is familiar with the basics, you can start to teach them more advanced commands. You will need to learn specific commands if you want to do agility with your dog. These tips will help you have fun with your dog, and to see his potential. If you are looking to have a competitive relationship with your dog, these tips will be a great foundation for training.

Teach your dog how to fetch

Fetch is a great game to play with your dog. It can be hard to believe that your dog might not want to play fetch or don't understand the rules. Fetch is a natural game for some dogs, especially sporting dogs and hounds. It can also be easier to teach than others. For others, like toy dogs and other small dogs, fetch is a foreign concept. It is possible to teach it. Dogs will love fetch for hours once they get the hang of it.

These are some tips for teaching your dog to fetch

* It may be necessary to start from scratch when teaching your dog to chase objects. Start by waving the object to your dog until he grabs it. Reward him once he takes the object in his mouth. Keep doing this until he associates the act of picking up an object with a treat. Next, throw it a few feet away. Once you have taught him the association between the object & the treat, he should start to chase it. If he succeeds, reward him by picking up the object. Continue practicing until your dog is comfortable chasing the object. Do not rush this step. Take your time and help your dog to understand the "chase" idea.

* Next, get your dog to bring the object back to you. To get him to come back, you can use the 'Come!' command. If this doesn't work and he continues to stare blankly at you and is far away with the object in hand, you can show him another toy or wave it in front of him. You will get him used to coming back to you when you throw an object for him. Continue practicing until he comes back with the first object. Praise him when he does.

* Tell him to drop the object and then show him the second. Reward him for dropping the first object. Continue practicing until he can drop the object by hearing "Drop" and without actually seeing it.

*Some dogs will run off when they catch an object. It can be hard to get them back. If this sounds familiar to your dog, you can teach your dog "fetch" on a leash. This exercise may require a long leash. Your dog can throw the object as far as the leash will allow and then let it go. To encourage your dog to return to you when he has caught it, pull gently on the leash.

Reward him when he comes back to you. These steps should be repeated until he realizes that he should return to you after chasing. He will eventually get the hang of it.

Sometimes the problem is that the dog may come back and drop the object. When this happens, you can say "bring it back" and encourage your dog to pick up the object again. It may take patience but once your dog does it, praise him and reward him with a treat to keep him going. Make sure you're using toys that your dog enjoys. It will be difficult to get your dog to chase sticks if he doesn't show any interest. It is a good idea to use his favorite toy as a starting point.

Teaching the Command "Place"

This skill is useful for dogs to learn. It will teach your dog how to wait at a specific place. This is useful in situations where guests arrive at your home and your dog becomes anxious. To calm your dog, you can use the word 'Place' to command him to stop barking and go to a designated place. Your dog must be able to respond to the commands 'Sit' or 'Stay' before you can teach this skill.

Put the leash on your dog, and say the word "Place" or any other word you like. You can lead your dog to the place you want him to go by saying the word. Give him a treat once he's there. You can continue practicing the leash many times before you give up and go without it. You can give him the leash off if he doesn't understand it. If that happens, you can just keep practicing until he gets the hang of it. When he is able to understand and go to his place, you can command him to either sit or lie down. Before giving him a treat, make sure he remains down for at least 10 seconds. Continue practicing until he is able to stay put for at least two to three minutes.

Asking To Go Outside

Your dog may already have a routine for toileting. Your dog might need to go at a different time than normal, even though you may have a strict schedule. It would be great if your dog could let you know when he wants to go.

You can teach him how to use the outside toilet.

These are the steps:

Hang something that makes a loud noise next to your dog's door. This will be the place you go to when you take your dog to the bathroom. It should be secure and low enough that your dog can reach it.

* Toys with bells are a good choice. It is best to not hang it on the dog's door. It will ring each time you go outside, sending mixed signals to your dog.

* After you have done this, start to ring the bells whenever you go outside with your dog to use the toilet. This will help you associate toilet breaks with the ringing bells.

* Reward your dog for touching the bells or sniffing them before you leave the house. This will help him to make the connection between the bells and his business.

* Reward this behavior until he can touch the bells every time he uses the toilet. He will touch the bells to let you know if he has to go.

Teaching the Command "Heel"

To teach your dog heel, he should walk next to you with your leg while you walk. This will help you keep your dog calm and under control. If you are going to compete in agility or other competitions with your dog, it is a crucial skill. Stand still and have your dog stand next to you in order to teach "Heel". Your dog should be standing right next to you, looking in the same direction. You can say firmly, "Heel", and then take a few steps forward. Your dog should follow you and be right next to your leg. You can reward him for doing this and increase the distance you walk together.

It isn't always easy to teach 'Heel'. A training collar or leash may be needed to help your dog learn and understand what you expect. Research the best training collars for your dog. You can also use a heel stick to get your dog to walk along with you.

To reward your dog's good behavior, give him a treat when he walks to heel.

How to get your dog to stop barking

Barking is an instinctive form of communication that dogs use to alert them of dangers or intruders. Sometimes barking can go beyond this and may be a result of bad habits or unintentionally being conditioned to bark. This is annoying but can be overcome with patience and understanding.

First, don't shout at him. You may think he is barking at you, and if he does that, a shout can cause him to get even more excited. Don't try and stop him by soothing his ears. This can be understood by you sending a positive signal that will encourage him to bark more.

There are many ways to stop your dog from barking. A head halter can be used to force your dog's mouth shut when he barks. It isn't cruel and doesn't cause any harm. This is an easy way to manage unwanted barking. When he stops barking, praise him. You can also distract him from the problem by giving him distractions. He will startle you by slapping a magazine on the table. You can reward him if he stops.

Sam Parker, a Jack Russell cross, was my friend. He was perfect in every way except barking. "Bruce would bark at anything. The wind, the postman, and the neighbor's cat. Sam said that everything was possible. He was more encouraged by my shouting, so I placed a folded magazine at the table. Every time he cried for nothing, I would smash the table. He would be shocked and I would reward him. He was still vocal for a while, but now he's calmer and more confident.

Other dog tricks

It's not just a way to impress your guests or friends with dog skills, but it can also be a great way for you to have fun and bond with your dog. These are some other tricks that you can teach your dog:

* Bark on Command Encourage your dog to bark when you say 'Speak' or "Bark", and reward him when he does.

* Shake the Paw. This is a simple trick to teach, especially if you have treats in your hands. If they are unable to get the treat through their mouths, your dog will naturally give you their hand. You can make it so they give you their paw while you say "Give me Your Paw" or "Paw". This is how to make it happen.

If they do, you should reward them.

* Roll over. * Roll Over. Next, use the command "Roll" and encourage your dog to roll over by giving him a treat.

The Key Takeaways

This chapter will discuss some of the more difficult commands that you can teach your dog. These commands will give you an idea about what your dog can do, as well as how to train it to stop undesirable behavior. You will need to teach your dog advanced skills if you plan to compete with him. This can make it so much more fun for you both.

* We covered advanced commands like fetch, place, ask for the outside, heel, and stop barking.

* You should not practice advanced commands until your dog is proficient in the basics. It will take patience. But the rewards will be worth it!

We will be discussing how to properly care for your dog in the next chapter.

Conclusion

Dogs are influenced by their instincts. Dogs respond to stimuli based on their perception of it. The most aggressive behavior results from the perception and protection of one's territory, values and position in the family hierarchy.

Both genetic and environmental factors can both contribute to aggression. Training your dogs is one way to reduce aggression. There are some things you should and shouldn't do when training your dogs. Your dogs will be most grateful if you are patient, consistent, and kind to them. Aggressive behavior, which includes punishing and encouraging violent behavior, can only be reinforced by being aggressive.

www.ingramcontent.com/pod-product-compliance
Lightning Source LLC
Chambersburg PA
CBHW070101120526
44589CB00033B/1242